Chancelier Cirimwami

Shortage of drinking water in South Kivu, risk of cholera epidemic

Chancelier Cirimwami

Shortage of drinking water in South Kivu, risk of cholera epidemic

Contribution to the study of the risks of a cholera epidemic linked to the shortage of drinking water (Kadutu health zone)

ScienciaScripts

Cover image: www.ingimage.com

This book is a translation from the original published under ISBN 978-620-6-72406-3.

Publisher:
Sciencia Scripts
is a trademark of
Dodo Books Indian Ocean Ltd. and OmniScriptum S.R.L publishing group

120 High Road, East Finchley, London, N2 9ED, United Kingdom
Str. Armeneasca 28/1, office 1, Chisinau MD-2012, Republic of Moldova, Europe
Printed at: see last page
ISBN: 978-620-8-16172-9

TABLE OF CONTENTS

EPIGRAPH

"Research is the future, but reading teaches, informs, guides, directs, leads and enriches".

DEDICATION

This work is dedicated to all readers who wish to awaken their sense of knowledge and enrich their self in a lasting way by strengthening their awareness.

THANK YOU

Our thanks to the Lord Almighty for his blessings during our study.

This work would not have been possible without the cheating contributions of those who took part in the data collection.

We would particularly like to thank the people who gave us their precious time and who enriched this work with their criticisms, comments, suggestions and guidance.

We would also like to thank the management team of the KADUTU health zone for their unconditional collaboration.

To all those who, from near or far, have participated in the realisation of this work and whose names have not been mentioned, may they find in this work the mark of our gratitude.

SUMMARY

Introduction: Cholera is a key indicator of poor socio-economic development and a threat to public health worldwide. We conducted this study with the aim of describing the risks of a cholera epidemic in the Kadutu health zone following a shortage of drinking water.

Methodology: This was a cross-sectional descriptive study conducted from May 2024 to August 2024. The sampling was simple random, which included 385 people, the data were collected by KoboCollect and analysed in Epi Info 7.2.

Results: A total of 385 people were interviewed, all of whom were informed about cholera, its sources, modes of transmission, signs and means of prevention. The source of information was the media (76.1%), followed by 18.96% of community intermediaries, with 51.43% confirming insalubrity and lack of hygiene as the source, 59.48% mentioning diarrhoea and dehydration as signs, and 44.68% mentioning compliance with hygiene and sanitation measures as a means of preventing the disease.

94.81% of respondents confirmed shortages in their living environments, and 96.88% said that water-borne diseases occur during shortages, especially in the dry season. This population is therefore at greater risk of catching cholera because of the shortage of water and the lack of mechanisms to purify the water from standpipes and ponds that will be used by the communities.

Conclusion: The issue of sanitation is a major factor in preventing cholera, as is the application of other essential measures to combat it. It is vital that the political and health authorities step up to the plate to tackle this scourge, which is slowly decimating the population.

Key word : Risk, Epidemic, Cholera, Shortage

INTRODUCTION

1. ISSUES

Cholera is an acute diarrhoeal infection, the severe form of which is characterised by extreme watery diarrhoea rapidly leading to potentially fatal dehydration. The infection is caused by ingestion of food or water contaminated with the *Vibrio cholerae* bacillus. Although it can be easily treated with oral rehydration salts, cholera remains a global threat due to its high morbidity and mortality in populations, especially vulnerable ones with insufficient access to adequate healthcare.(WHO, 2017)

The year 2022 saw an acceleration of the 7^{e} cholera pandemic, with a doubling in the number of cases notified to the WHO worldwide compared with 2021 (472,697 cases compared with 223,370) and an increase in the number of countries reporting cases, from 35 in 2021 to 44 in 2022. The geographical distribution of cholera epidemics has also changed: some countries that had not recorded cholera cases for many years, such as Lebanon and the Syrian Arab Republic, were affected by major outbreaks in 2022. Very large outbreaks, characterised by the presence of more than 10,000 suspected or confirmed cases in a given country, were reported by 7 countries on 2 continents (Afghanistan, Cameroon, Malawi, Nigeria, Syrian Arab Republic, DRC and Somalia). The number of very large outbreaks has more than doubled compared with each of the previous years.(WHO, 2023)

Worldwide, men and women were affected in equal proportions, with a male/female ratio of 1. However, some countries reported an unequal gender distribution, which may reflect differences in risk factors.

In 2022, 9 European countries reported a total of 51 cases (47 of which were imported) and zero deaths. Although European countries have the water, sanitation and hygiene services and health systems needed to rapidly contain transmission of the disease, the number of imported cases is a reminder that there is a risk of cholera spreading worldwide from any active outbreak of the disease(WHO, 2023).

In the Middle East and Asia, 16 countries reported 372,205 cases of cholera and 394 associated deaths (case-fatality rate of 0.1%) in 2022. Of these cases, 56 were imported; 4 countries reported only imported cases (Bahrain, Kuwait, Singapore, United Arab Emirates). In addition, 17 countries reported 0 cases. The regional distribution of cases in 2022 differed significantly from that in 2021. Yemen reported no cases in 2022, whereas it accounted for

89% of the region's cases in 2021. Two of the countries reporting outbreaks, Lebanon and the Syrian Arab Republic, had not recorded a case of cholera for more than a decade(WHO, 2023). Afghanistan accounted for 77% of cases and 34% of deaths reported in the region; all cases from this country were reported as suspected cases. Afghanistan and the Syrian Arab Republic reported a high proportion of cases in children under 5 years of age (55% and 45%, respectively). Overall, Asia recorded an increase in the number of diarrhoeal disease outbreaks in 2022(WHO, 2023).

In Africa, 17 countries had reported 100,437 cases of cholera and 1955 deaths (case-fatality rate of 1.9%), including 202 imported cases in 2022. In addition, 13 countries had reported 0 cases. This represents a 29% drop in the number of cases and a 52% drop in the number of deaths reported compared with 2021; the case-fatality rate has fallen from 2.9% to 1.9%. This apparently favourable trend should, however, be interpreted with caution. In 2021, Nigeria was hit by a very large-scale epidemic, accounting for 78% of cases and 88% of deaths reported in Africa("Weekly Epidemiological Record" Relevé Épidémiologique Hebdomadaire 2023).

In other countries, the number of notified cases has more than doubled, from 30,055 in 2021 to 76,598 in 2022, and the number of reported deaths has increased 2.5-fold, from 490 in 2021 to 1,358 in 2022(WHO, 2023).

In 2022, the geographical dispersion of cases and deaths was greater than in 2021, and no single country reported more than 25% of cases or 30% of deaths. Five African countries reported very large outbreaks with more than 10,000 cases (Cameroon, Malawi, Nigeria, DRC and Somalia)(WHO, 2023).

Africa has seen an exponential increase in the number of cholera cases against a backdrop of a sharp rise in cases worldwide. The number of cases notified on the continent in the first month of 2023 alone has already reached more than 30% of the total number of cases recorded for the whole of 2022.(WHO, 2022)

By 29 January 2023, an estimated 26,000 cases and 660 deaths had been reported in 10 African countries affected by epidemics since the start of the year. In 2022, around 80,000 cases and 1,863 deaths had been recorded in 15 countries affected by cholera. If the current rapid upward trend continues, the number of cases could exceed that recorded in 2021, which was the worst year for cholera in Africa in almost a decade. The average case-fatality rate, currently close to 3%, is higher than the 2.3% achieved in 2022 and well above the acceptable threshold of less than 1%.(WHO, 2022)

Since the beginning of 2024, on 18 February, the number of cholera cases and deaths reported to the WHO Regional Office for Africa was 40,115 and 965 respectively, with a case-fatality rate of 2.4%. DRC, Ethiopia, Mozambique, Zambia and Zimbabwe accounted for 95.7% (38,397) of total cases and 97.1% (937) of total deaths this year (Pierre A et al 2017).

The DRC is currently reporting regular outbreaks of this scale, mainly in endemic provinces in the east of the country.
In 2023, from the beginning of the year to epidemiological week 48, the Democratic Republic of Congo had recorded more than 48,280 suspected cases of cholera, including 421 deaths. North Kivu, one of the six provinces where the WHO has activated a UN-mandated scale-up of its emergency operations, has alone reported around 62% of the country's cholera cases, against a backdrop of massive population displacement and poor coverage in terms of drinking water and hygienic latrines, particularly in the camps for internally displaced people around Goma. This has made it one of the worst epidemics in the country's recent history since 2017(WHO, 2023).

From the beginning of 2024 to epidemiological week 8, 7,774 suspected cases of cholera, including 158 deaths (case-fatality rate 2.0%), were notified across 74 health zones belonging to 9 provincial health divisions. At the end of S08/2024, 1,083 cases and 9 deaths (case-fatality ratio 0.8%) were reported in 34 health zones, with no substantial change in the number of cases compared with the previous week (1,081 cases and 21 deaths: case-fatality ratio 1.8%). Overall, the case-fatality rate fell between S07 (1.8%) and S08 (0.8%). The provinces of North Kivu (740 cases) and Haut Katanga (187 cases) account for almost all (927 cases: 85.2%) of the cases reported in the country. (John, Rick et al 2006).

In South Kivu, cases are reported every year in both rural and urban areas. More than 70 cases of cholera were reported in the space of a week, from 14 to 20 May 2023, in the town of Bukavu. According to the South Kivu provincial health division, the Kadutu health zone is the worst affected, with 49 cases, followed by Bagira and Ibanda, with 17 and 5 cases respectively. (DPS, 2023)

In the city of Bukavu, the Kadutu health zone recorded the most cases, and the consumption of dirty water and the shortage of water in Bukavu are at the root of this epidemic.(DPS, 2023).

Research questions

- What are the risks of a cholera epidemic in the Kadutu health zone as a result of the shortage of drinking water?

Objectives

General objective

Describe the risks of a cholera epidemic in the Kadutu health zone as a result of the shortage of drinking water.

Specific objectives

- Identify the factors that may contribute to the occurrence of cholera in the urban health zones of Bukavu in general and Kadutu in particular.
- Evaluate the level of case management received in cholera treatment centres and other health facilities in the Kadutu health zone

2. INTEREST OF THE SUBJECT

Personal interest

In addition to these objectives, which are the scientific focus of this research, we found that the population of the Kadutu health zone was concerned about the resurgence of cholera cases and the hygiene and sanitation situation in their environment.

We therefore decided to carry out this research to find out what cases had occurred and what kind of behaviour was characteristic of the population. We visited several families where the lack of hygiene and sanitation was thought to be at the root of health problems.

Scientific interest

This study could serve as a frame of reference for anyone interested in the problem of cholera and how to prevent it throughout the province of South Kivu and the Kadutu health zone in particular.

3. DELIMITATION OF THE SUBJECT

This subject is limited in time and space

It will be carried out over a period running from April to June 2024.

The study will be carried out in the KADUTU urban health zone,

4. METHODOLOGICAL APPROACH

For this study, we used a literature review and a retrospective survey as our methodological approach.

5. BRIEF PRESENTATION

Apart from the introduction and conclusion, this work is divided into four chapters, including :

- Chapter 1: REVIEW OF THE LITERATURE
- Chapter 2: METHODOLOGY
- Chapter 3: PRESENTATION OF RESULTS
- Chapter 4: DISCUSSION

CHAPTER ONE: LITERATURE REVIEW

1.1. THEORETICAL REVIEW

Definition of concepts

Risk: Possible danger that is more or less foreseeable

Epidemiology: is a scientific discipline which studies health problems in human populations, their frequency, distribution in time and space, and the factors influencing health and disease in populations.

Epidemic: a disease that affects a large number of people at the same time and in the same place.

Cholera : Cholera is an acute diarrhoeal infection caused by ingestion of food or water contaminated with the bacterium *Vibrio cholerae* (Taty B 2022).

GENERAL INFORMATION ON CHOLERA

Cholera is an acute diarrhoeal infection caused by the ingestion of food or water contaminated with the bacterium *Vibrio cholerae*. Cholera remains a global threat to public health and an indicator of a lack of equity and insufficient social development.

Vibrio cholerae strains

There are many serogroups of *V. cholerae*, but only 2 serogroups, O1 and O139, are responsible for outbreaks. The majority of recent outbreaks are due to *V. cholerae* O1, while O139, first identified in Bangladesh in 1992, has caused outbreaks in the past, but is now only identified in sporadic cases and remains confined to Asia. The disease caused by both serogroups remains the same (Pierre A et al. 2017).

Transmission modes

The transmission of cholera is closely linked to poor environmental management. The disease develops in environments where minimum drinking water and sanitation requirements are not met. It is therefore an indicator of inadequate development.

Contamination is oral and of faecal origin.

Direct transmission :

- Consumption of contaminated water or food.

- Direct contact with an infected person: sweat, which is rich in vibrios, plays an important role in human-to-human transmission, especially in dry tropical areas.
- Exposure to the excrement or vomit of an infected person.

Indirect transmission

Certain arthropods, mainly flies, play a role as vectors in the spread of vibrios.

Symptoms

Cholera is an extremely virulent disease that is transmitted by ingesting contaminated water or food. It can cause severe acute watery diarrhoea and, if left untreated, severe forms of the disease can kill within hours.

Most people infected with *V. cholerae* show no symptoms, although the bacillus is present in their faeces for one to 10 days after infection and is eliminated into the environment, where it can potentially infect other people.

For those who do develop symptoms, they are mild to moderate in the majority of cases. Symptoms appear between 12 hours and five days. In a minority of patients, acute watery diarrhoea develops, accompanied by severe dehydration. If left untreated, this can lead to death (Pierre A et all, 2017).

Epidemiology, risk factors and burden of disease

In epidemiological terms, cholera can be endemic or epidemic.

A cholera-endemic region is an area where confirmed cholera cases have been detected for three of the last five years, with local transmission established (meaning that cases are not imported). An outbreak/epidemic can occur both in endemic countries and in countries where cholera does not usually occur.(A. Dimandja, 2022)

There is a close link between cholera transmission and inadequate access to drinking water and sanitation facilities. Typically, places at risk include peri-urban shanty towns, as well as camps for internally displaced people or refugees.

Humanitarian crises, which in particular result in the interruption of water supply and sanitation systems and the displacement of populations into poorly equipped and overcrowded camps, can increase the risk of cholera transmission, if the bacillus is ever present or if it is introduced. There have never been any reports of epidemics involving the corpses of uninfected people.(Taty B, 2022)

Prevention and control

A multi-pronged approach is essential to combat cholera and reduce mortality. The measures used combine surveillance, improved water supply, sanitation and hygiene, social mobilisation, treatment of the disease and oral cholera vaccines.

Monitoring

Cholera surveillance should be part of an integrated disease surveillance system that includes local feedback and global exchange.

Cases of cholera are detected on the basis of a presumptive clinical diagnosis in patients aged two and over presenting with acute watery diarrhoea and severe dehydration, or dying as a result of acute watery diarrhoea.

Rapid diagnostic tests (RDTs) can be useful in detecting cholera outbreaks; however, to confirm the diagnosis, stool samples are sent to a laboratory for confirmation of the presence of *V. cholerae* O or O139 by bacterial culture or PCR (polymerase chain reaction) testing.

Surveillance for a cholera outbreak involves reporting patients suffering from acute watery diarrhoea and carrying out regular tests on a subset of these patients.

Local capacity to detect and monitor (collect, compile and analyse data) cases of cholera is essential to ensure the effectiveness of the surveillance system and to plan control measures.

Cholera-affected countries are advised to strengthen disease surveillance and national preparedness to rapidly detect and respond to potential outbreaks. Under the International Health Regulations, notification of all cholera cases is no longer mandatory. However, public health events involving cholera must still be assessed against the criteria set out in the Regulations to determine whether official notification is required (WHO, 2023).

Treatment

Cholera is easy to treat. Most sufferers can be cured by rapid administration of oral rehydration salts (ORS). The standard sachet of ORS is dissolved in 1 litre (l) of drinking water. Up to 6 litres of ORS may be needed to treat moderate dehydration in an adult patient on the first day.

Severely dehydrated patients present a risk of shock, and rapid administration of intravenous fluids is essential. These patients also receive appropriate antibiotics to shorten the duration of the diarrhoea, reduce the quantities of rehydration fluid required and shorten the duration of excretion of *V. cholerae* bacilli in their faeces.

All patients should start eating ordinary local food prepared safely as soon as it is safe to do so.

Breastfeeding should also be encouraged. Rapid access to treatment is essential during a cholera outbreak. Oral rehydration must be available in communities, including specific oral rehydration points, and not just in larger health centres that can offer intravenous infusions and treatment at any time. With rapid and appropriate treatment, the case-fatality rate should remain below 1%.

Zinc is an important adjunctive treatment for children under the age of 5. It also reduces the duration of diarrhoea and can prevent subsequent episodes of acute watery diarrhoea due to other causes.

Outlook

The global roadmap to 2030 comprises 3 strategic areas:

1. Early detection and rapid response to contain outbreaks: the strategy focuses on containing outbreaks wherever they occur through early detection and a rapid multisectoral response, with community involvement, strengthening surveillance and laboratory capacity, preparing health systems and supplies, and supporting rapid response teams;

2. A targeted multisectoral approach to prevent a resurgence of cholera: the strategy calls on countries and partners to focus on "hotspots", the relatively small areas most affected by the disease, where transmission can be interrupted by improving the supply of drinking water, sanitation and hygiene, and by administering OCV;

3. An effective coordination mechanism covering technical support, advocacy, resource mobilisation and partnership at local and global levels. The Task Force provides a solid framework to help countries scale up their cholera control efforts, based on country-led, cross-sectoral programmes and providing the necessary human, technical and financial resources.

In May 2018, the Seventy-first World Health Assembly adopted a resolution to promote the prevention and control of cholera and to endorse the document entitled "Ending Cholera: A global roadmap to 2030".

1.2. EMPIRICAL REVIEW

Gbary AR and Dossou JP conducted a descriptive and analytical cross-sectional study on the epidemiological and medico-clinical aspects of the cholera epidemic in the Littoral department of Benin in 2008. The aim of the study was to identify the epidemiological and medico-clinical characteristics of the cholera epidemic in the Littoral department of Benin in 2008. Methods. The study was based on 404 patient records, including information on patient identity, clinical and therapeutic aspects, and course of the disease. Ten randomly selected patients participated in a focus group discussion. The authorities in charge of managing the epidemic and health workers were interviewed in depth. Ten affected neighbourhoods were visited. The average age of patients was 23.72 ± 14.80 years. Attack rates by district ranged from 15.86 to 172.98 cases per 100,000 inhabitants. The Agbodjèdo, Hlacomey and Enagnon districts had significantly higher attack rates than the other districts. The case-fatality rate was 0.24%.

The endemicity of cholera in Cotonou can be explained by the massive uncontrolled occupation of the banks of the lagoon, combined with inadequate basic sanitation and difficulties in supplying drinking water. Vibrio cholerae O:1 was found in 19 of the 36 stool samples. The strains were all sensitive to ciprofloxacin, but resistant to cotrimoxazole. Diarrhoea was constant, 88.11% of cases vomited and 39.35% were severely dehydrated. Oral rehydration, parenteral rehydration and antibiotic therapy were used in 99.50%, 85% and 97.77% of cases respectively. Patients were treated with doxycycline for adults and amoxicillin for pregnant women and children. The length of stay at the treatment centre was significantly longer for patients with severe dehydration (Bampangue Ed 2022).

1.3. LOGICAL FRAMEWORK FOR THE RESEARCH

1.3.1. CONCEPTUAL FRAMEWORK

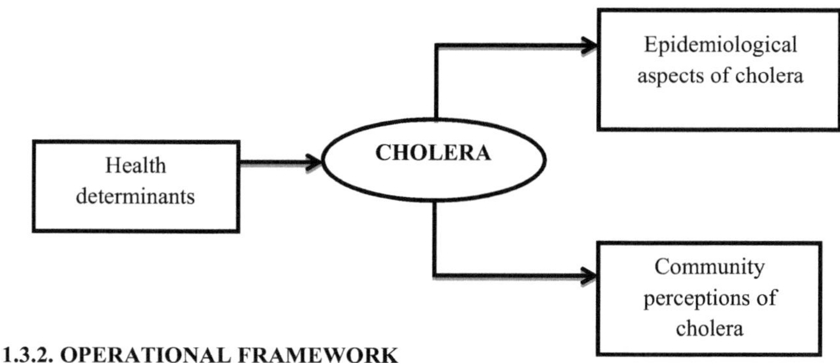

1.3.2. OPERATIONAL FRAMEWORK

We proceeded by documenting in libraries and on the internet, then writing the first part, then developing the interview guide followed by the survey, followed by the encoding of the data collected and discussion and the handing in of the work after corrections.

1.3.3. DEFINITION OF STUDY VARIABLES

Dependent variable

In this study, the dependent variable was the cholera epidemic.

Independent variables

As independent variables, we selected the epidemiological risks of cholera in the Kadutu health zone.

CHAPTER TWO: METHODOLOGY

2.1. STUDY SITE

The Kadutu health zone is one of 34 health zones in the province of South Kivu, and is an urban area with a population of 429,505.

Health situation

The Kadutu Health Zone currently has the following health facilities: Five 2e level facilities, including: the Dr RAU CIRIRI General Reference Hospital and the KADUTU General Hospital, the Bukavu University Clinics (MUHANZI), the Saint Vincent Medical Centre and the CBCA NYAMUGO Hospital Centre. The KADUTU Health Zone has two specialist centres: the SOSAME Psychiatric Centre and the HERI KWETU Rehabilitation Centre for the Disabled, as well as 12 health centres out of the 15 required, representing 80% health coverage. These are the MARIA, NEEMA, CBCA NYAMUGO, UZIMA, SOS, FUNU, 8e CEPAC, Mgr KATALIKO, Mgr MULINDWA, CECA 40, MAENDELEO, CIRI health centres.

Table 1. Total population of the Kadutu HZ in 2024 by health area

N°	Health areas	Total population
1	BINAME	36567
2	BUHOLO 2	31846
3	CECA MWEZE	32589
4	CIMPUNDA	34048
5	CIRIRI I	60646
6	CIRIRI II	22922
7	FUNU	26390
8	LURHUMA	21525

9	**MARIA/KARHALE**	**79257**
10	**NEEMA**	**24403**
11	**NYAMUGO**	**29842**
12	**NYAMULAGIRA**	**25537**
13	**UZIMA**	**16834**
TOTAL		442 406

Geographical location

The Z.S of Kadutu is an integral part of the city of Bukavu. It is located in the commune of Kadutu, with a surface area of 15km² and a population density of 21120 inhabitants per km².

It is limited :

To the north by the river Wesha, which separates it from the BAGIRA Health Zone

To the south-east by the River KAWA and the main road of the Avenue Industrielle, which separates it from the IBANDA Urban Health Zone.

To the west by a conventional boundary at CISIRWE, which separates it from the KABARE rural health zone.

To the south-west by the villages of LUGUSHA and NYAMIERA, which separate it from the NYANTENDE Health Zone.

It has a mountainous terrain and a humid mountain climate, with an average temperature of 15°C in the rainy season and 25°C in the dry season. It is situated at an altitude of 1462 m. Its longitude is between 28° 50'E and -2°30' S. Its vegetation is wooded savannah.

2.2. TYPE OF STUDY

This was a descriptive, cross-sectional study designed to contribute to the study of the risks of a cholera epidemic following a shortage of drinking water in the Kadutu health zone.

2.3 MATERIAL

We used a survey questionnaire via the SMART PHONE

2.4. SAMPLING

We used simple random sampling for the population of the Kadutu health zone

Sample size

We used the Schwartz formula to determine the sample size

$$n = \frac{Z\propto^2 * p * q}{d^2}$$

Z = 1,96
p = 50% = 0,5
q = 50% = 0,5
d = 0,05

$$\mathrm{n} = \frac{(1{,}96)^2 * 0{,}5 * 0{,}5}{(0{,}05)^2} = \frac{3{,}8416 * 0{,}5 * 0{,}5}{0{,}0025} = \frac{0{,}9604}{0{,}0025} = \mathbf{384{,}16 \approx 385}\ \boldsymbol{sujet}\ \text{à}\ \boldsymbol{enqueter}$$

2.5. DATA COLLECTION METHODS AND TOOLS

We conducted a survey using the Kobo Collect application

2.6. DATA COLLECTION PLAN

We will conduct a survey using a survey questionnaire

2.7. TREATMENT AND ANALYSIS PLAN

To assess the results, we used SPSS software to represent the data in frequency tables and graphs.

2.8. ETHICAL CONSIDERATIONS

We reassured the respondents that the information they provided would be kept confidential, while respecting their anonymity and their informed consent and choice.

2.9. STRENGTHS AND LIMITATIONS OF THE STUDY

Forces

- This study provides decision-makers with clear and important information to guide them in their health decisions.
- Clarification of the real questions that have long remained unanswered, and this is the originality of this wide-ranging subject by providing

Limits

- The unavailability of sufficient and relevant theories for a better understanding of cholera.

PRESENTATION OF RESULTS

Table I. Distribution of respondents by socio-demographic characteristics

Variables	N	%
Age of respondent		
Under 25	80	20,78
26 to 35 years	113	29,35
36 to 45 years	149	38,7
Over 45s	43	11,17
Gender		
Male	179	46,49
Female	206	53,51
Type of respondent		
Father	94	24,42
Mother	133	34,54
Child	158	41,04
Level of study		
Primary	33	8,57
Secondary	200	51,95
University	152	39,48
Profession (occupation)		
Student	92	23,90
Civil servant	88	22,86
Contractor	53	13,77
Humanitarian	2	0,52

Unemployed	89	23,11
Salesperson	61	15,84
Civil status		
Single	166	43,12
Married	203	52,73
Widower	16	4,15
Size of your household		
Less than or equal to 5	142	36,88
More than 5	243	63,12
Religion		
Catholic	229	59,48
Protestant	111	28,83
Muslim woman	15	3,90
Kimbanguist	3	0,78
Jehovah's Witnesses	27	7,01
Total	**385**	**100**

The table shows that the majority of respondents were aged between 36 and 45, and more than half were women, married and had a primary education. In terms of occupation, students were in the majority, followed by the unemployed, 6/10 of whom lived in households of more than 5 people, with Catholicism and Protestantism being the predominant religions.

Table II. Distribution of respondents by residential environment

Variables	N	%
Length of time in the neighbourhood		
Less than a year	67	17,4
1-3 years	106	27,54
More than 3 years	212	55,06
Total	**385**	**100**
Toilet type		
With fake	271	70,39
Without false	114	29,61
Total	**385**	**100**
Availability of a water supply on the plot		
Available at	150	38,96
Not available	235	61,04
Total	**385**	**100**
Source of water supply		
Neighbour's tap	124	52,77
Fountain bollard	111	47,23
Total	**235**	**100**

From this table, we can see that more than half the respondents had lived in their plot for more than 3 years, with 7/10 of households having a false toilet, while more than 6/10 of households did not have a source of water in their plot, with more than half getting their water from neighbours and the rest from standpipes in the **area.**

Table III. Distribution of respondents according to information on cholera

Variables	N	%
Information on cholera		
Informed	385	100
Source of information		
Media	293	76,1
Community relay	73	18,96
Social networks	19	4,94
Understanding the causes of cholera		
Know	385	100
The causes of cholera		
Eating poorly washed or unprotected raw food	59	15,32
Not washing your hands before eating	16	4,16
Drinking untreated water	71	18,44
Failure to wash hands after using the toilet	41	10,65
Insalubrity, rubbish, lack of hygiene	198	51,43
Knowledge of the signs of cholera		
Know	385	100
Signs of cholera		
Diarrhoea and dehydration	229	59,48
Vomiting and fatigue	117	30,39
Lack of appetite	39	10,13
Knowledge of how to prevent cholera		
Know	385	100

How to prevent cholera		
Use of clean latrines	51	13,25
Drink clean water	64	16,62
Eat food that is well cooked and protected	58	15,06
Eat fruit and vegetables washed in clean water	40	10,39
Compliance with hygiene and sanitation measures	172	44,68
Total	**385**	**100**

This table shows that all respondents were informed about cholera, its causes, signs and means of prevention. More than ¾ of respondents had received their information from the media, followed by community relays. In terms of causes, insalubrity was the most common, and more than half confirmed diarrhoea and dehydration as signs of cholera, while compliance with hygiene and sanitation measures was the most common way of preventing cholera.

Table IV. Distribution of respondents according to attitudes to cholera

Variables	N	%
What to do if cholera occurs		
Drink ORS and go to hospital	246	63,89
Quick access to a CTC or health centre	139	36,11
Total	**385**	**100**
Behaviour in the event of contact with a cholera patient		
Don't tell anyone	4	1,04
Disinfecting yourself	80	20,78
Heading for a CTC	301	78,18
Total	**385**	**100**
Dealing with a person cured of cholera		
Stay away from him	216	56,1
Getting close to him	169	43,9
Total	**385**	**100**

Reading this table, we see that over 6/10 of respondents supported the attitude of drinking ORS and then going to hospital, and over ¾ supported the option of going to a CTC in the event of contact with a cholera patient, while over half said they would not go near a patient who had recovered from cholera.

Table V. Distribution of respondents by water shortage situation

Variables	N	%
Water shortages by district		
It happens	365	94,81
It doesn't happen	20	5,19
Total	**385**	**100**
Occurrence of disease during water shortages		
It happens	373	96,88
It doesn't happen	12	3,12
Total	**385**	**100**
Number of cases of illness during shortages		
A case	144	38,61
Two cases	101	27,07
Three cases	76	20,38
Four cases or more	52	13,94
Total	**373**	**100**
How to avoid cholera		
Use of water and clean latrines	106	27,53
Hand washing with soap or ash	148	38,44
Compliance with hygiene rules	131	34,03
Total	**385**	**100**
The seriousness of cholera		
It's a serious illness	385	100
Risk of cholera during water shortages		

Lower risk	22	5,71
High risk	363	94,29
Total	**385**	**100**
Possibility of eradicating cholera in Kadutu		
It can be done	385	100

The table shows that more than 9/10 of respondents confirmed that shortages can lead to cholera and other waterborne diseases in their neighbourhoods, with the majority reporting having recorded a case of illness linked to the shortage. All respondents confirmed the seriousness of cholera and the possibility of eradicating the disease.

DISCUSSION OF THE RESULTS

Cholera, the disease caused by *Vibrio cholerae*, is one of those scourges which, in the collective unconscious, seem ancient but are still very much with us today.

Cholera is therefore a very recent phenomenon in Africa. Its history dates back to the early 1970s with the 7th pandemic, which began in 1961 in the Sulawesi archipelago in Indonesia. Since 1970, several cholera epidemics have been reported in several African countries, including the Democratic Republic of Congo.

The aim of this study was to describe the risks of a cholera epidemic in the Kadutu health zone following the shortage of drinking water.

This health zone is one of the areas of the province affected by this epidemic. This sharp rise in the number of cases is making the population, and their visitors, more vulnerable to cholera.

A total of 385 people residing in the Kadutu health zone were included in the results of this study, of whom 20.78% of the respondents were aged less than or equal to 25 years, 29.35% of those aged between [26 - 35 years], 28.7% of those aged between [36 - 45 years] and 11.17% aged over 45 years, 28.7% of those aged between [36 - 45] and 11.17% over 45. As for marital status, 52.73% were married, 43.12% single and 4.15% widowed. Of these, we found that a higher proportion were women (55.51%) than men (46.49%), with 8.57% having primary education, 51.95% secondary education and 39.48% university education. As for religious beliefs, 59.48% were Catholics, 28.83% Protestants, 3.9% Muslims, 0.78% Kimbanguists and 7.01% Jehovah's Witnesses. In terms of occupation, 23.9% were students, 22.86% civil servants, 13.77% entrepreneurs, 0.52% humanitarians, 15.84% shopkeepers and 23.11% unemployed, compared with the study by Amos Kamundu on the knowledge, attitudes and practices of the population of the Mugunga health area, on preventive measures against cholera: In the Karisimbi health zone, which aimed to describe the knowledge, attitudes and practices of the population on cholera prevention measures in the MUGUNGA health area, a total of 653 respondents made up the results of the study, including 6.6% of respondents in the 41 and over age group, 44.1% in the 31 to 40 age group, 45.32% in the 21 to 30 age group and 3.98% in the 10 to 20 age group. 69.67% of respondents were married, 15.16% single, 8.8% widowed and 6.27% divorced. In terms of occupation, 34.6% of respondents worked in small businesses, 30.93% were housewives, 12.55% were farmers, 9.8% had no occupation, 3.21% were fishermen, 2.29% were teachers, 2.75% were civil servants, 1.83% were health workers and 1.99% were in other occupations. In terms of level of education, 15.92% of respondents had higher education/university, 56.04% secondary education, 19.75% primary education and 8.26% no education, of whom 25.11% were men and 74.88% women.(Amos KAMUNDU, 2013). The results of the study on the knowledge, attitudes and practices of mothers of children under the age of 5 regarding diarrhoeal diseases in the Lukonga health zone in the city of Kananga show that the most represented age group is 26-31, with 28.7%. The average age is 29 plus or minus a standard deviation of 7, with 63% of people living in couples and 37% single. In terms of level of education, 52% of respondents had secondary education, followed by primary education (20%), university education (18%) and no education (10%). The results show that 66.7% of respondents were unemployed or housewives, followed by employees or managers (25.3%) and those in the informal sector (8%).(Albert et al. 2024)

As for the nature of the respondents, 24.42% were fathers, 34.54% were mothers and 41.04% were sons and daughters. 63.12% of households had more than 5 people and 36.88% had less than or equal to 5 people. In terms of household size, many of the households lived in overcrowded conditions, which exposed them to serious health problems, including cholera, as compared to the study on the knowledge, attitudes and practices of the population of the

Mugunga health area, on measures to prevent cholera: Karisimbi health zone, which aimed to describe the knowledge, attitudes and practices of the population on cholera preventive measures in the MUGUNGA health area, shows that the majority or 83, 15% of respondents have 3 or more children(Amos K., 2013)

Our study shows that 55.06% of respondents had lived in their respective areas for more than 3 years, 27.54% for between 1 and 3 years and 17.4% for less than a year. 70.39% of respondents used toilets with faults and 29.61% used those without faults. As for the availability of a source of water in their plot, 61.04% had stated that it was not available, while 38.96% had a source of water, of which 2 sources were raised for those who did not have a source of income, 52.77% obtained their water from neighbours' taps and 47.23% from standpipes, comparing this with the studies. A comparison with the knowledge, attitudes and practices of mothers of children under the age of 5 about diarrhoeal diseases in the health zone of lukonga, city of kananga, shows that 51.3% of mothers rely on rainwater, 30% on river water and 14% on tap water; 3.3% borehole water and 1.3% water from a standpipe, while 84.7% of respondents did not treat water at home, compared with 15.3% who did.(Albert et al. 2024)These behaviours put children at much greater risk of diarrhoeal diseases, including cholera.

In this study, all respondents had information on cholera, its causes, signs, modes of transmission and prevention, with the majority (76.1%) mentioning the media as a source of information, followed by community relays (18.96%) and social networks (4.94%). Most of the respondents (51.43%) said that the causes of cholera were unhygienic conditions, followed by 18.44% who said that drinking dirty, untreated water and 15.32% who said that eating raw and/or badly washed, unprotected food was the cause. In terms of signs, 59.48% confirmed diarrhoea and dehydration, (30.39%) vomiting and fatigue and 10.13% a lack of appetite. In terms of means of preventing cholera, 44.68% confirmed compliance with hygiene and sanitation measures, 16.62% for drinking clean water and 15.06 for eating well-cooked and protected food, compared with the results of the study on the knowledge, attitudes and practices of the population of the Mugunga health area, on cholera prevention measures: In the Karisimbi health zone, **the** majority of respondents (98.77%) said they had already heard of cholera, 36.14% of them from community relays. Of these, 22.1% knew that drinking non-potable water was a cholera transmission route, 3.8% knew that rubbish was present in the environment and 32% knew that eating without washing hands was a cholera risk factor. It emerged that 54.51% of our respondents knew that rice-like stools were a sign of cholera and 18.83% knew that vomiting was a sign of cholera. As for prevention, 42.57% of respondents knew that washing their hands with soap or ash and using clean water were measures to prevent cholera, 27.41% were in favour of covering food properly, 10.71% were in favour of having hygienic toilets and 19.29% were in favour of avoiding contact with suspected cases of cholera.(Amos K., 2013). In comparison with the results of the study on the knowledge, attitudes and practices of mothers of children under the age of 5 about diarrhoeal diseases in the health zone of Lukonga, city of Kananga, 67% of respondents had already heard about diarrhoeal diseases, 36% of whom had heard about them through the media, 25.3% through community intermediaries, 24% through medical staff and finally 24% through the health services; 24% from medical staff and 14% from neighbours. As symptoms of diarrhoea, 61.2% of respondents cited dehydration, followed by fatigue (26.9%). The others mentioned fever (8.6%) and finally those who mentioned convulsions or neurological disorders (3.2%).(Albert et al. 2024)

In terms of attitudes, 63.89% agreed to drink ORS and go to hospital in the event of cholera, and 36.11% agreed to go quickly to a CTC or health centre.

Attitude in case of contact with a cholera patient: 78.18% go to a CTC, 20.78% disinfect and 1.04% say nothing. In the case of contact with a person recovered from cholera, 56.1% chose not to approach and 43.9% chose to approach.

As far as attitudes are concerned, it is important to raise awareness of cholera in terms of the attitudes to adopt.

With regard to the water shortage, 94.81% agreed that there was a water shortage in their neighbourhoods, and 96.88% agreed that diseases occur during water shortages, especially water-borne diseases, and 38.61% agreed that they had developed cholera during a shortage. All respondents agreed that cholera was serious and could be eradicated, 94.29 did not agree that a cholera carrier could be asymptomatic, while in the study on the knowledge, attitudes and practices of mothers of children under 5 on diarrhoeal diseases in the health zone of Lukonga, 81% of our respondents their children had suffered from diarrhoea against 19% whose children had not suffered from diarrhoea.

Cholera has major economic and sociological consequences, including reduced production, exports and tourism. It is therefore imperative to improve living conditions for the population, to strengthen epidemiological surveillance and to involve the population in programmes to combat cholera and other water-borne diseases.

Particular emphasis should be placed on hygiene measures and the development of health education:

Raising public awareness,

Water supply in sufficient quantity (minimum 20 litres per person per day) and quality (water chlorination, protected water points, adequate sewage disposal system),

Sanitation and hygiene: control of excreta (latrines) and waste (rubbish pits), distribution of soap, control of markets, burial of corpses,

Curative measures: treatment in a Cholera Treatment Centre includes, in addition to ORS or infusion therapy, disinfection of patients (hands and skin) with a 0.05% chlorine solution; disinfection of homes, bedding, stretchers, cooking utensils, clothing and transport vehicles with a 0.2% chlorine solution; disinfection of latrines, excreta, cadavers and foot baths with a 2% chlorine solution.

Cholera remains a major but neglected public health threat. It is a challenge for the international community, requiring the involvement of everyone to eradicate it.

CONCLUSION

At the end of the study, which focused on "Contributing to the study of the risks of a cholera epidemic following the shortage of drinking water in the Kadutu health zone", the company announced that it would be conducting a study on the risk of a cholera epidemic in the Kadutu health zone.

The results of the study point to a high level of knowledge about cholera, in terms of causes, signs, modes of transmission, means of prevention and attitudes to adopt when cholera occurs. Added to this are the factors likely to explain the high rate of water-borne diseases, including cholera, i.e. the shortage of water in this health zone, as well as non-compliance with hygiene and sanitation measures.

Compliance with hygiene and sanitation measures is the key to beating this disease in the Kadutu health zone, especially during the dry season, when there is an upsurge in cases of water-borne diseases.

These results argue in favour of stepping up information and awareness-raising campaigns on the fight against cholera, improving the supply of drinking water in South Kivu province and urban planning standards, as well as treatment for cholera and other water-borne diseases. The DRC has committed itself to putting an end to cholera, by opting for the roadmap to 2030 via a global partnership. This commitment is proof of the efforts underway in the country to strengthen the health sector.

RECOMMENDATIONS

To the health authorities of South Kivu

1. Continue awareness-raising campaigns, particularly aimed at people living in urban areas, reassuring them of the benefits of cholera prevention, while at the same time dispelling the prejudices surrounding knowledge of cholera.
2. Involve pre-trained community workers.
3. Monitor and evaluate the recommended hygiene and sanitation activities.
4. Making drinking water supplies available
5. Raising awareness of health and hygiene standards
6. Do everything possible to minimise the risk of cholera.

To the public

1. Compliance with hygiene and sanitation measures.
2. Get your water from clean, designated sites for quality water
3. Boil water to the recommended degree before use
4. Use of certain antiseptic products recommended for quality assurance, in particular chlorine, ...

BIBLIOGRAPHICAL REFERENCES

1. Albert et al. 2024 ; Connaissances, attitudes et pratiques des meres des enfants de moins de 5 ans sur les maladies diarrheiques dans la zone de sante de LUKONGA, ville de KANANGA/ KASAI CENTRAL/ RD CONGO",
2. Ndié J, Bayoro I, Takoukam I, Wina P, Wina P. Étude Des Aspects Épidémiologiques Du Choléra Dans Le District De Santé De Tchollíré (Nord- Cameroun).
3. Camacho A, Bouhenia M, Alyusfi R, Alkohlani A, Naji MAM, de Radiguès X, et al. Cholera epidemic in Yemen, 2016-18
4. Gbary AR, Dossou JP, Sossou RA, Mongbo V MA. Epidemiological and medico-clinical aspects of the cholera epidemic in the Littoral department of Benin in 2008.
5. Boutin J, Delva GG, Mabou MM, Pape JW, Peck M, Wright PF, et al. Importance of Cholera and Other Etiologies of Acute Diarrhea in Post-Earthquake Port-au-Prince, Haiti. Am J Trop Med Hyg.

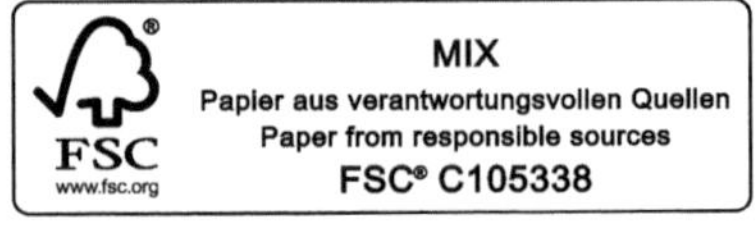

Printed by Books on Demand GmbH, Norderstedt / Germany